FIRST TIME EXPECTANT

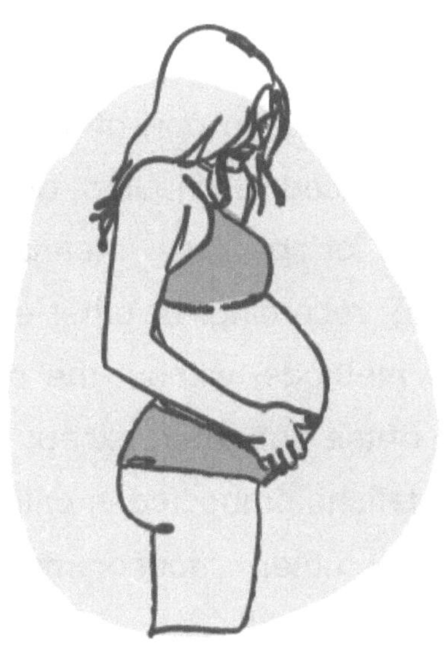

Ultimate Guide for New mum and Dad

ANNA BROWN

Forward

Becoming a parent for the first time is a profound transition filled with joy, anticipation, and perhaps a hint of uncertainty. This book aims to be a trusted resource, offering insights, guidance, and shared wisdom to support you through each stage of this remarkable voyage.

From the initial excitement of pregnancy to the magical first days at home with your newborn, we explore the emotional landscape, provide practical tips, and celebrate the unique bond between new parents and their little ones. Throughout, the emphasis is on embracing the journey, fostering a strong partnership, and finding joy in the everyday moments of parenthood.

Anna, a soon-to-be first-time mom, eagerly awaited the arrival of her baby. Amid the anticipation and occasional nervousness, a thoughtful friend gifted her a book titled "First

Time Expectant: New Dad and Mum." Little did Anna know that this simple gesture would become a beacon of support and guidance throughout her parenthood journey.

As her due date approached, Anna delved into the book, finding solace in its pages. The comprehensive advice on setting up the nursery, preparing for labor, and navigating the emotional roller coaster of new parenthood became her go-to guide. Anna particularly appreciated the emphasis on the importance of communication and shared responsibilities with her partner, Mark.

When the big day arrived, Anna and Mark faced labor with newfound confidence, armed with insights from the book. The couple found strength in each other, understanding the process and navigating the challenges with a shared sense of purpose. The book's practical tips on newborn care and postpartum adjustments proved invaluable during those initial days at home.

As the weeks unfolded, Anna and Mark encountered various parenting challenges, but the book provided a reassuring voice, offering connecting with other parents sharing similar experiences, strategies for balancing work and family, coping with sleep deprivation, and navigating postpartum changes.

Months later, Anna reflected on the transformative impact the book had on her parenting journey. The well-thought-out advice, personal anecdotes, and expert insights not only helped her navigate the practical aspects of parenthood but also provided emotional support during moments of uncertainty. The book became a cherished companion, offering wisdom and encouragement as Anna and Mark celebrated the milestones of their baby's first year.

In the end, "First Time Expectant: New Dad and Mum" became more than just a gift – it became a trusted friend, guiding Anna and

Mark through the beautiful chaos of parenthood and enriching their experience in ways they never imagined.

As you embark on the incredible journey of parenthood, this guide warmly welcomes you to the transformative experience awaiting both new moms and dads. In these pages, you'll find not just practical advice but a compassionate companion to navigate the thrilling, challenging, and heartwarming moments that parenthood brings.

Whether you're seeking advice on setting up the nursery, navigating the challenges of postpartum life, or simply craving reassurance during those sleepless nights, this guide is crafted with care to be a reliable companion.

Parenthood is a shared adventure, and as you turn these pages, may you find comfort, inspiration, and a wealth of knowledge to empower you on this extraordinary voyage into the world of new beginnings.

Congratulations on this exciting chapter in your lives, and may it be filled with boundless love, growth, and the immeasurable joy that parenthood brings.

Warm regards,
Anna Brown
Author.

PREFACE

Welcome to "First Time Expectant: New Dad and Mum." In these pages, we embark on a shared journey into the remarkable world of parenthood. As the author, my aim is to offer a guide that goes beyond the conventional and delves into the heart of the transformative experience that is becoming a parent for the first time.

This book is not just a collection of advice; it's a companion for those exhilarating yet challenging moments, a source of comfort during the sleepless nights, and a roadmap for navigating the uncharted territory of new parenthood. Drawing from a blend of personal experiences, expert insights, and the shared wisdom of countless parents, I crafted this guide with the hope that it becomes a valuable resource for you as you welcome the newest member of your family.

Parenthood is a journey that unfolds uniquely for each individual, yet it's a collective experience that binds us together. From the excitement of the

positive pregnancy test to the tender moments of holding your newborn for the first time, every chapter of this book is designed to provide guidance, encouragement, and a sense of camaraderie.

As you flip through these pages, you'll discover practical advice on setting up the nursery, insights into navigating the emotional landscape of pregnancy and postpartum, and reflections on the evolving partnership between new moms and dads. The emphasis is not only on surviving but thriving in the adventure of parenthood.

This book is dedicated to every expectant parent seeking reassurance, knowledge, and a touch of inspiration. Whether you find comfort in shared experiences, practical tips, or the celebration of milestones, may this guide accompany you on your unique journey, turning moments of uncertainty into opportunities for growth and joy.

Here's to the incredible adventure of becoming parents for the first time – may it be filled with love, laughter, and the discovery of the extraordinary in the ordinary. my aim is that readers will get information for best their best practice

Dedication

This book is dedicated to all Expectant parents in the world

TABLE OF CONTENT

Introduction

In the quiet anticipation of new life, where the air is charged with the promise of tiny fingers and baby coos, we find ourselves at the threshold of one of life's most transformative journeys – the journey of becoming a first-time expectant parent. It's a path marked by exhilarating highs, tender moments, and the occasional flutter of nervousness, all woven into the tapestry of new beginnings.

As the author of "First Time Expectant: New Dad and Mum," I invite you to embark on this voyage with me. Whether you're a mom-to-be, a dad eagerly awaiting fatherhood, or a couple navigating the uncharted waters together, this book is crafted to be your companion through the myriad emotions, challenges, and joys that define the path to parenthood.

The pages ahead unfold a narrative that is both universal and deeply personal. Drawing from shared experiences, expert insights, and the collective wisdom of parents who have walked this road before, we explore the nuanced landscape of expectant parenthood. From the initial thrill of the positive pregnancy test to the tender moments in the nursery, each chapter is designed to offer not just advice but a sense of camaraderie – a reminder that you are not alone on this extraordinary journey.

In these pages, we'll delve into practical considerations, from setting up the nursery to navigating the intricacies of labor and delivery. Yet, beyond the practicalities, we'll also explore the emotional terrain – the shared responsibilities, the evolving partnership between new moms and dads, and the indescribable bond that forms as you cradle your newborn for the first time.

"First Time Expectant" is more than a guidebook; First child expectant is a celebration of the significant transformation of becoming a parent brings. Whether you're seeking insights into the challenges that lie ahead, tips for self-care during the whirlwind of early parenthood, or simply a moment of connection with the experiences of others, this book is here to accompany you.

As we embark on this journey together, I am convinced that this pages is a source of comfort, knowledge, and inspiration, guiding you through the adventure of a lifetime – the adventure of welcoming your first child into the world.

Mark and I, a couple deeply in love. our cozy home echoed with laughter and shared secrets, and as we gazed into the future, the idea of starting a family began to blossom in their hearts.

Pregnancy Preparations:

As we decided to embark on the journey of parenthood, we eagerly dove into the world of pregnancy preparations. our weekends transformed into a whirlwind of nursery shopping, baby clothes picking, and discussions about the perfect shade for the baby room. we attended parenting classes, read countless books on pregnancy, and discovered the joy of planning for the arrival of their little one.

Anna, myself, meticulous by nature, created detailed lists of baby essentials, from cribs to onesies, while mark my husband, the ever-supportive partner, painted the nursery walls with hues of soft pastels. Together, we navigated the sea of advice from experienced parents, seamlessly blending the practical aspects of preparation with the warmth of shared dreams.

Conception and Early Pregnancy:
our journey took a momentous turn when I discovered I was pregnant. The positive test

was met with tears of joy, hugs that lingered a little longer, and the overwhelming realization that our lives were about to change forever. As the news settled, we couple experienced a profound shift in connection, a shared understanding that a new chapter was unfolding.

The early stages of pregnancy brought a mix of emotions. I navigated morning sickness with a smile, supported by mark's gentle care and endless cups of ginger tea. we attended doctor's appointments together, marveling at the ultrasound images that gradually transformed a tiny blob into a recognizable human form. The baby's heartbeat became a rhythmic melody, the soundtrack to their shared excitement and anticipation.

The Journey to Birth:
As the months passed, my belly swelled with the promise of new life. we couple attended

childbirth classes, where we learned about breathing techniques, labor positions, and the art of being each other's anchor during the birthing process. The due date approached, and our home became a hub of preparation – bags packed, nursery perfected, and the car seat installed with meticulous care.

When the day arrived, contractions painted the canvas of anticipation. mark stood by my side, offering words of encouragement and unwavering support. In the delivery room, our bond deepened as we faced the challenges of labor together. my strength mirrored by mark's reassuring presence, and with each passing moment, we couple drew closer to the miracle awaiting them.

Welcoming the Newborn:
In my hushed serenity of the delivery room, the cries of our newborn filled the air, and we became parents. The journey that began with

whispered dreams had now materialized into the soft, tangible weight of their daughter nestled in mark's arms. Tears of joy flowed freely as we marveled at the perfection of this tiny being, a culmination of love, hopes, and dreams.

The initial days at home were a dance of sleepless nights and tender moments. we both embraced the challenges of newborn care with a shared commitment. Late-night feedings became a sacred ritual, and diaper changes transformed into opportunities for whispered lullabies. we navigated the roller coaster of emotions, finding solace in our shared responsibility and the unspoken bond that grew stronger with each passing day.

Conclusion:
And so, in the embrace of family and the warmth of a loving home, myself, mark and the newborn daughter embarked on the adventure

of a lifetime. Parenthood, with its challenges and joys, unfolded before us , a journey marked by shared laughter, whispered secrets, and the boundless love that comes with the miracle of creating a family. As they gazed into the eyes of our little one, mark and I knew that the story of their journey had just begun, a story written in the delicate strokes of everyday moments and the profound magic of parenthood.

let journey Together…

PART 1

Conception: Pregnancy Journey

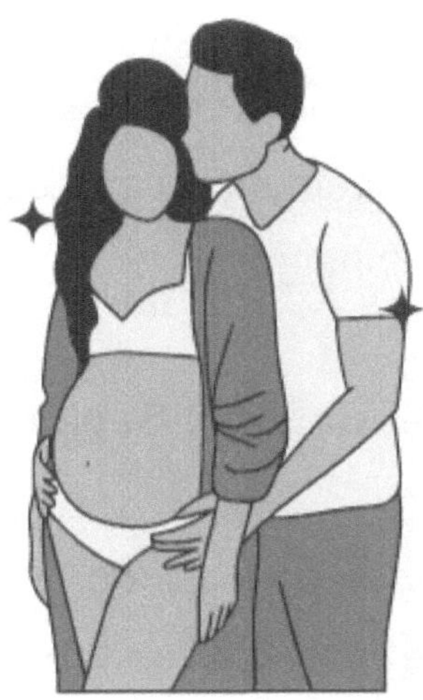

starting the parenthood journey

i. *Anticipating Parenthood*

In the quiet moments before parenthood, as the sun sets on one chapter of life and rises on another, there exists a unique and delicate space filled with the anticipation of the extraordinary journey ahead. For couples awaiting the arrival of their first child, this period is akin to standing at the threshold of an unexplored realm, where every heartbeat and flutter of excitement resonates with the promise of new beginnings.

The Promise of New Beginnings:

Anticipating parenthood is a profound experience that weaves dreams, hopes, and a dash of nervous excitement into the fabric of everyday life. It's a time when conversations shift from mundane routines to the nursery colors, baby names, and the shared vision of what it means to become a family. Each positive pregnancy test, doctor's appointment, and ultrasound becomes a chapter in the unfolding story of a family in the making.

The promise of new beginnings is painted in the soft hues of nursery walls and the meticulous selection of baby clothes. It's the whispered conversations about parenting philosophies and the unspoken commitment to face the unknown together. The journey begins with the realization that life, as they know it, is about to transform into something beautiful and unknown.

There are unexpected pregnancies. Congratulations if you're among the women who randomly took a pregnancy test after feeling nauseous and were pregnant.

research shows that married between 35 and 39 were about 90 percent as likely to have a child as those who got married younger than 35; women who got married between 40 and 44 years old were only about 62 percent of conception, and women who got married between 45 and 49 were only 14 percent. Stated differently, only approximately 14% of people who married after 45 had children, but almost everyone who married between 20 and 35 had at least one child compared to that of those who got married at 45.

it's true that it is hard to get pregnant at old age but not impossible. The more you look for data on internet where we have lots of junks and writers , you will get confused and also read old datas, the more worried you would be. Just take your mind off age, stop focusing on getting older. instead channel your energy exercising and getting rest before getting pregnant.

Also, you need to be conscious of weight, cause lots of research have pointed that obesity makes getting pregnant difficult. Related research has shown a connection between obesity, infertility, and miscarriage. Maternal obesity is linked to poorer breastfeeding outcomes and a delayed onset of breast milk after delivery. If you are overweight, shelding some weight before pregnancy Will be a lot of Benefit.

Health and Technology keeps improving, so women will keep being fertility in the future.

Not long, I got the good news after 6 year... congratulations to me once again. lol."

How to get Pregnant

To get pregnant, you need a good Timing, you need sperm to be around , when egg is released during ovulation.

most female have a cycle of 28 days, measured from the start of each period to the start of the subsequent one. Day 1 is the beginning day of your menstrual cycle. Ovulation preparation takes place the week before and the week after your period. The release of the egg, known as ovulation, occurs about 14 days following the onset of your period and it starts its descent towards the uterus.

During this time, egg is produced, these egg which is reading available for fertilisation then travel, which takes a few days. if the egg come into contact with a sperm while traveling towards the uterus,it will cause fertilisation to takes place.
if you get lucky to release two eggs and both meet sperm, you get twins.
Twins may additionally occur if the fertilised egg divides precisely at the starting point. Upon fertilization of the egg (or eggs) arrives in the uterus, implantation takes place, and actually the start of pregnancy. The method starting with an egg

Six to twelve days pass between release and implantation. For the majority of healthy pregnancies, implantation takes place between

22 and 24 days following your last menstrual cycle's first day.

The luteal phase is the entire second half of the cycle that occurs after the egg is released. Depending on whether you become pregnant, this phase is either occupied with fertilisation and implantation, or it is spent with the egg remaining in the uterus until it is flushed out during your menstrual cycle. Your period will arrive on day 28 if you are not pregnant. Should you become pregnant, your period will end on day 28 and you'll be set to go. This is the general schedule (for an individual with a typical 28-day cycle; if your cycle is longer or shorter, you may ovulate before or after day 14).

The sperm must be waiting for the egg to begin its journey down the tube, which is essential to pregnancy. This indicates that the day before or the day of ovulation is the ideal time for insemination or sexual activity. Sperm take some time to swim into the fallopian tubes, hence typically the day following ovulation is too late.

However, sperms Usually, can survive for up to five days in the
fallopian tube, waiting. This indicates that the window is in actuality a little bit longer. 4–5 days prior to ovulation, having sex can lead to a baby, although it's less common.

why does it still takes time to get pregnant. we know fully well that most couples trying to get babies have sex alot. then why?
 There are some ways to dictate ovulation for right timing, the most common are;
Cervical mucus and Basal body temperature (BBT).

Basal body temperature (BBT).-When they wake up each day and before they start any activity, women who are interested in finding out when they are fertile should take their oral, vaginal, or rectal temperature. The recording features of contemporary digital thermometers make BBT monitoring easier.

The interpretation of BBT might take several forms. One way, called the "coverline" method, involves drawing a horizontal coverline, or threshold temperature, on a BBT chart. Ovulation is suggested when a temperature is reported over this cutoff line.

The most affordable way to identify ovulation is by cervical mucus. Women might use their fingers to gather vaginal mucus or they can just observe the mucus that is visible at the vulva.

Cervical mucus is been secreted by cervical and endocervical glands. Cervical mucus can emerge at different times during the menstrual cycle. This mucus' primary ingredient, high-molecular-weight glycoprotein (mucin), produces a mesh-like structure that acts as a barrier to sperm and microorganisms outside of the periovulatory phase. Inspection reveals the mucus to be viscous, sparse, and thick. Oestrogen has the effect of increasing acellular water production and decreasing mucin formation throughout the periovulatory period. As a result, the mesh-like structure relaxes and opens up significantly for sperm entry.18, 39, 40 During this time, women tend to discharge more watery material that looks like raw egg white.

The symptothermal approach refers to the combination of monitoring BBT and examining cervical mucus for contraception.

There are ovulation Dictection kits now .

Navigating Emotions:

Amidst the joyous anticipation, there exists a tapestry of emotions – excitement, nervousness, and perhaps a touch of anxiety. The realization that roles are about to evolve, responsibilities will multiply, and sleep might become a precious commodity can be both thrilling and daunting. Anticipating parenthood is a delicate dance between acknowledging the changes that lie ahead and embracing the unknown with open hearts.

For many, this period is marked by self-reflection and the exploration of personal and shared values. It's a time to assess one's own upbringing, consider parenting styles, and envision the kind of home they want to create for their child. The shared dreams and expectations become the foundation upon which the journey into parenthood unfolds.

Building Connection:

As the due date approaches, anticipating parenthood becomes a journey of building connection. Partners find solace in each other's company, discovering new layers to their relationship as they navigate the unknown territory together. Communication becomes a lifeline, allowing couples to share fears, dreams, and the small joys that come with awaiting the arrival of their little one.

From attending prenatal classes to reading parenting books together, the couple begins to craft their unique approach to parenthood. The shared laughter, late-night conversations, and quiet moments of reflection deepen the connection between partners, creating a sense of unity that will serve as the cornerstone of their family.

Embracing the Journey:
In the gentle cadence of awaiting parenthood, there is an invitation to embrace the journey rather than merely anticipate the destination. It's about savoring the present, celebrating the small milestones, and finding joy in the anticipation itself. The baby kicks, the nesting instincts, and the shared glances of excitement become the soundtrack to this extraordinary chapter of life.

As the calendar pages turn, the couple steps into the realm of parenthood, not as experts but as enthusiastic explorers. The anticipation, once a quiet undercurrent, bursts forth into the kaleidoscope of the first cry, the touch of tiny fingers, and the overwhelming love that fills the room when they finally have their newborn arrival.

And so, the journey begins – a journey that transcends the anticipation and unfolds into the magical tapestry of parenthood, where every moment, from the first flutter to the sleepy cuddles, becomes a cherished part of the story they are writing together.

you are pregnant, congratulations…

ii. Navigating the first Trimester

Navigating the First Trimester: A Compassionate Guide to the Beginnings of Pregnancy.

The first trimester of pregnancy unfolds as a delicate symphony of changes, both physical and emotional. As expectant parents embark on this transformative journey, navigating the initial weeks requires a blend of self-care, support, and an understanding of the unique challenges that accompany this remarkable period.

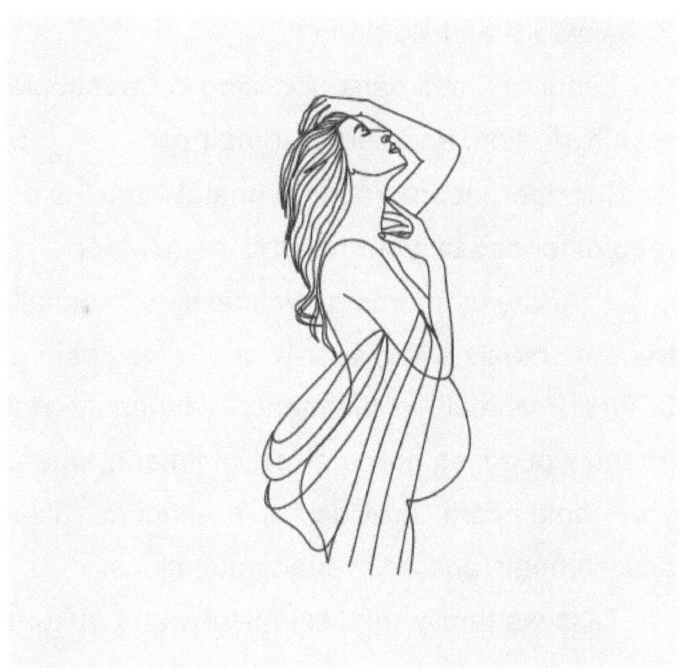

1. Confirmation and Embracing the News:

- Confirm the pregnancy with a visit to a healthcare provider.
Share the news with your partner and decide when and how to share it with close family and friends.

- Embrace the emotions that come with this revelation, allowing space for both excitement and any initial concerns.

2. Self-Care and Nutrition:

   - Prioritize self-care, focusing on adequate rest, hydration, and balanced nutrition.

   - Consider incorporating prenatal vitamins as recommended by your healthcare provider.

   - Address morning sickness with small, frequent meals and ginger-based remedies.

3. First Prenatal Appointment: -Schedule and attend your first prenatal appointment, where your healthcare provider will conduct initial assessments and answer any questions.

   - Discuss family medical history, and ensure open communication about any concerns or queries.

4. Emotional Support:

   - Establish open communication with your partner about your feelings and expectations.

   - Seek emotional support from friends, family, or online communities to connect with others experiencing similar emotions.

- Understand that mood swings are common due to hormonal changes, and consider engaging in activities that bring comfort and joy.

5. Managing Symptoms:

    - Be prepared for common symptoms like morning sickness, fatigue, and breast tenderness.

    - Experiment with different coping mechanisms, such as ginger tea for nausea or napping to combat fatigue.

    - Communicate openly with your healthcare provider about any severe symptoms or concerns.

6. Lifestyle Adjustments:

    - Review and, if necessary, adjust your lifestyle choices to prioritize the health of both you and your baby.

    - Minimize exposure to potential hazards, such as certain medications or environmental factors.

- Discuss with your healthcare provider any necessary modifications to your exercise routine.

7. Planning and Preparing:

- Begin researching childbirth and parenting options.

- Create a preliminary plan for maternity leave, discussing it with your employer if applicable.

- Start considering and researching baby essentials, such as cribs and strollers, to ease the later stages of preparation.

8. Regular Exercise:- Engage in moderate, pregnancy-safe exercises, such as walking or prenatal yoga.

- Consult your healthcare provider before starting or modifying any exercise routine.

9. Educate Yourself:

- Read reliable resources about pregnancy and the first trimester.

- Attend prenatal classes to gain insights into childbirth, baby care, and postpartum adjustments.

10. Communication with Healthcare Provider:

- Maintain regular communication with your healthcare provider, attending all scheduled appointments.

- Discuss any concerns, questions, or changes in your well-being promptly.

Navigating the first trimester is a journey of discovery, filled with unique challenges and the promise of new life. By prioritizing self-care, seeking support, and staying informed, expectant parents can approach this initial phase with confidence and a sense of anticipation for the chapters that lie ahead.

iii. Emotions and Expectations

Pregnancy is a kaleidoscope of emotions, a transformative journey that weaves joy, anticipation, and occasional moments of uncertainty into the fabric of everyday life. As expectant parents embark on this profound adventure, understanding the nuanced emotional landscape and managing expectations becomes essential for a positive and connected experience.

Joy and Excitement: The revelation of a positive pregnancy test often sparks overwhelming joy and excitement. Embrace and celebrate this initial surge of positive emotions, sharing the news with loved ones to amplify the joy.

Nervousness and apprehension are natural companions to the joy, especially for first-time parents. Acknowledge these feelings, recognizing that uncertainties are a part of the journey and seeking support from partners, friends, or healthcare professionals.

Physical Changes and Body Image: let be conscious that as the baby bump gets bigger, the body undergoes remarkable changes, expect a spectrum of emotions related to body image.
Communicate openly with your partner about these changes, focusing on the shared experience of creating life.

Emotional sensitivity and mood swings might result from hormonal fluctuations during pregnancy.Recognize these changes as normal and communicate your feelings to your partner, ensuring a supportive environment. Husband need to really understand and give good support.

Anticipation and Planning: Anticipation often accompanies the planning phase, from envisioning the nursery to selecting baby names.

Bonding with the Baby: Establishing an emotional connection with the unborn baby is a unique and personal experience.
Engage in activities that promote bonding, such as talking or singing to the baby, and involve your partner in these moments.

Managing Expectations of Parenthood
Expectations about parenthood may vary, and it's crucial to communicate openly about roles and responsibilities.
Attend prenatal classes together to gain insights into childbirth, parenting styles, and newborn care, aligning expectations with shared knowledge.

Coping with Uncertainty: Uncertainty is inherent in pregnancy, from health concerns to the unknowns of labor.

Develop coping strategies, such as mindfulness or seeking guidance from healthcare providers, to navigate moments of uncertainty.

Establish a strong support system, including friends, family, and healthcare professionals.

Share your emotions with your partner and loved ones, fostering an environment of understanding and empathy.

Embrace the pregnancy journey as a shared adventure, acknowledging that both partners may experience emotions differently.

Regularly check in with each other, fostering a connection that strengthens as you navigate the emotional landscape together.

The pregnancy journey is a tapestry of emotions, each thread contributing to the unique narrative of your family's story. By acknowledging and embracing the spectrum of feelings, and by fostering open communication, expectant parents can weave a foundation of support and understanding that enhances the joy and connection throughout this extraordinary chapter of life.

Preparing for Arrival :

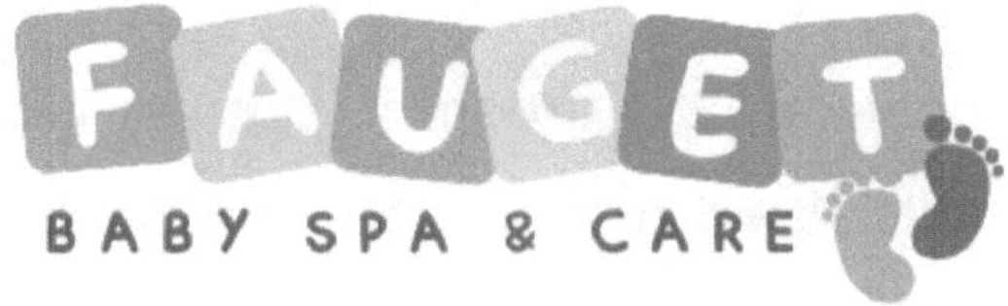

i. Setting Up the Nursery

As the days draw closer to the arrival of the little one, setting up the nursery becomes a beautiful journey filled with anticipation and love. choose a room or space, to be transformed into a haven where the dreams and the coos of the baby will echo.

In choosing the room, you envision the moments it will hold – the late-night feedings, the gentle lullabies, and the quiet giggles that will soon fill the air. Take your time to plan the layout thoughtfully, Choose a soothing color scheme for the walls. Opt for low-VOC paint to ensure a safe environment.

Decorate with soft furnishings, such as curtains, rugs, and wall art, to create a warm and inviting atmosphere considering every nook and cranny. The crib, with its promise of sweet dreams, found its place in a corner bathed in soft natural light. The changing table, adorned with cute little onesies, stands ready for the countless diaper changes and the giggles that may accompany them. And the comfortable chair by the window, a nook where stories will be read, and sleepy eyes will close in the warmth of embrace.

Ensure safety by Baby proofing the room by covering electrical outlets, securing furniture to the wall, and eliminating potential hazards.

Invest in storage solutions like shelves, baskets, and bins to keep baby essentials organized.

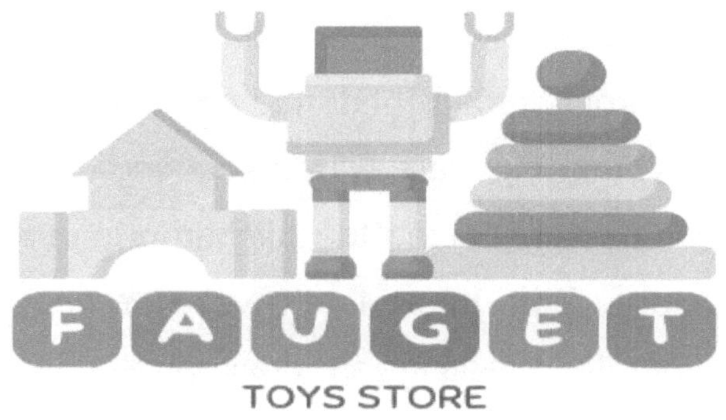

Label storage containers for easy access to diapers, wipes, clothing, and toys.Place a changing pad on top of the dresser or changing table.

Keep diapers, wipes, and diaper rash cream within arm's reach.

In choosing bedding and linens, Select comfortable and safe bedding for the crib, including a fitted crib sheet and breathable blankets.Have a few sets of crib sheets on hand for easy changes.

Don't forget to Install Proper Lighting, Use soft, adjustable lighting to create a calming environment for both daytime and nighttime activities. inConsider blackout curtains to control natural light during nap times.

Painting the walls with a soothing color palette was like choosing the backdrop to our family's story. Soft hues that evoke tranquility and warmth, creating an environment where the baby will feel safe and loved. It's a canvas waiting to be adorned with the artwork our little one will create and the pictures that will capture the essence of a growing family. The dresser, doubling as a changing table, is not just storage but a place where tiny socks and onesies will find their home. The shelves, adorned with books and toys, are an invitation to the wonders of imagination.

let your focus be creating a nurturing environment where the baby can explore, learn, and grow.The personalized touches will make the nursery uniquely yours. From the soft blankets to the framed photos and the little plush toys that already occupy a special place, the room is infused with our personalities and the love you feel for your little one.As you prepare to bring the baby into this world, the nursery stands as a testament of your love and readiness. It's a space that not only meets the practical needs of parenthood but is also a reflection of the dreams you hold for a growing family. With every gentle touch and every thoughtful decision, the nursery becomes more than just a room; it becomes a sanctuary of love, a cocoon where our family story unfolds.

Also, Set up and assemble essential baby gear, such as a bassinet, swing, or playpen, as needed.

For breastfeeding, create a comfortable feeding area with pillows and a side table for essentials.

Keep a small basket with snacks and water for yourself.

Ensure you have a supply of diapers, wipes, and other essential baby care items before your due date.

Invest in a trustworthy baby monitor so you can watch your child as they sleep.

Remember, the nursery is not just a practical space but also a reflection of your love and anticipation for your baby. Take your time, enjoy the process, and create a nurturing environment where you and your little one can thrive.

ii. *Baby Essentials Checklist*

Certainly, here's a general baby essentials checklist to help you prepare for your little one's arrival:

Clothing:

1. Onesies (short and long-sleeved)
2. Sleepsuits or footed pajamas
3. Baby hats
4. Socks or booties
5. Scratch mittens to prevent baby from scratching their face
6. Baby outfits for special occasions
7. Swaddle blankets or sleep sacks for sleep time

Feeding:

8. Bottles and nipples (even if breastfeeding, having some on hand can be helpful)

9. Breast pump (if breastfeeding)10. Nursing bras and pads

11. Formula (if not breastfeeding)

12. Bottle sterilizer

13. Bibs

14. Burp cloths

15. Nursing pillow

Diapering:

16. Diapers (consider newborn and size 1)

17. Baby wipes

18. Changing pad

19. Diaper rash cream

20. Diaper bag for outings

21. Diaper pail or disposal system

Sleeping:

22. Crib or bassinet

23. Crib mattress and fitted sheets

24. Waterproof mattress covers

25. Baby monitor

26. Swaddle blankets or sleep sacks

27. Pacifiers (if you choose to use them)

Bathing and Grooming:
28. Baby bathtub
29. Baby shampoo and wash
30. Soft baby towels
31. Baby hairbrush and comb
32. Nail clippers or baby scissors
33. Baby lotion or oil

Health and Safety:
34. Infant car seat
35. Stroller or baby carrier
36. First aid kit (thermometer, baby-safe pain reliever, nasal aspirator)
37. Baby-safe laundry detergent
38. Baby-safe cleaning products
39. Outlet covers and baby-proofing supplies
40. Smoke and carbon monoxide detectors in the house

Nursery and Furniture:

41. Crib and mattress

42. Changing table or dresser with changing pad

43. Rocking chair or glider

44. Storage for baby clothes and essentials

45. Nightlight or soft lighting for nighttime feedings

Clothing and Laundry:

46. Baby hangers

47. Baby laundry basket or hamper

48. Baby-friendly laundry detergent

Entertainment and Development:

49. Soft baby toys and rattles

50. Play mat or baby gym

51. Books for newborns and infants

52. Music or lullaby player

Remember, every baby is unique, and your specific needs may vary. This checklist is

based on your preferences and circumstances.
Happy nesting!

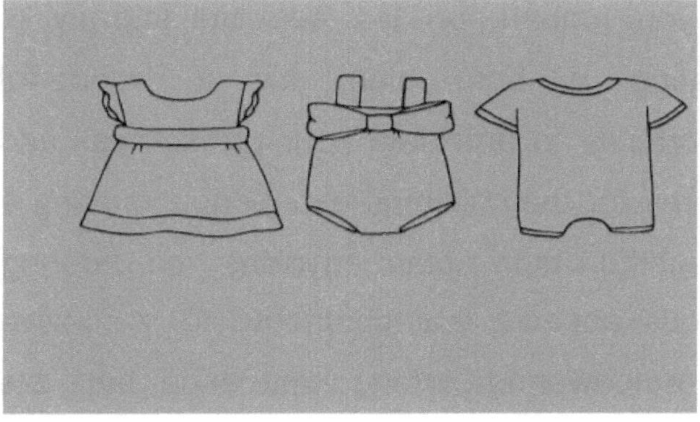

iii. Birth Plan Considerations

As you embark on the beautiful journey of creating a birth plan, it's a wonderful opportunity to articulate your preferences and desires for the childbirth experience. crafting a thoughtful birth plan involves considering various aspects that contribute to a positive and empowering birthing experience. here are some considerations to guide you:

1. communication and shared decision-making:
   - Being open and honest with your healthcare practitioner is essential. discuss your birth plan early in your pregnancy and be receptive to their expertise and guidance.
   - clearly express your preferences while remaining open to flexibility based on the progression of labor and medical considerations.

2. labor environment:

- consider the ambiance of the labor room. would you like soft lighting, music, or specific scents to create a calming atmosphere?

- decide who you'd like to be present during labor, whether it's your partner, family members, or a doula.

3. pain management:

- outline your preferences for pain relief options, whether it's natural pain management techniques, epidural anesthesia, or a combination.

- specify if you have specific preferences for movement, positions, or water immersion during labor.

4. monitoring and interventions:

- discuss your preferences for continuous or intermittent fetal monitoring during labor.

- outline your stance on interventions such as episiotomy, vacuum extraction, or forceps use. clearly communicate your preferences and any circumstances under which you would be comfortable with these interventions.

5. delivery preferences:

- specify your preferences for the birthing position and whether you'd like to use a birthing stool, squat bar, or other aids.

- express your preferences for guided pushing versus allowing your body to guide the process.

6. immediate postpartum period:

- consider your preferences for immediate skin-to-skin contact with your baby.

- outline your stance on delayed cord clamping and whether you'd like to bank cord blood.

7. cesarean section:

- while none of us hope for complications, consider your preferences in case a cesarean section becomes necessary.

- discuss preferences for partner presence in the operating room, immediate skin-to-skin contact, and any other postoperative considerations.

8. feeding preferences:
- specify your intentions regarding breastfeeding or formula feeding.
- if you plan to breastfeed, communicate your desire for assistance and support in the early postpartum period.

9. cultural or spiritual considerations:
- if there are cultural or spiritual practices you wish to incorporate into the birthing experience, communicate these to your healthcare team.

10. postpartum care and rooming-in:
- discuss your preferences for rooming-in with your baby and your partner staying with you in the hospital.

- outline any specific requests for postpartum care, including preferences for pain management and recovery.

remember, your birth plan is a guide, not a rigid script. it's a tool to help communicate your preferences, foster open communication with your healthcare team, and contribute to a positive birthing experience. be flexible, trust the expertise of your healthcare providers, and embrace the beautiful journey that lies ahead.

wishing you a safe and empowering birthing experience.

SUPPORTING EACH OTHER:

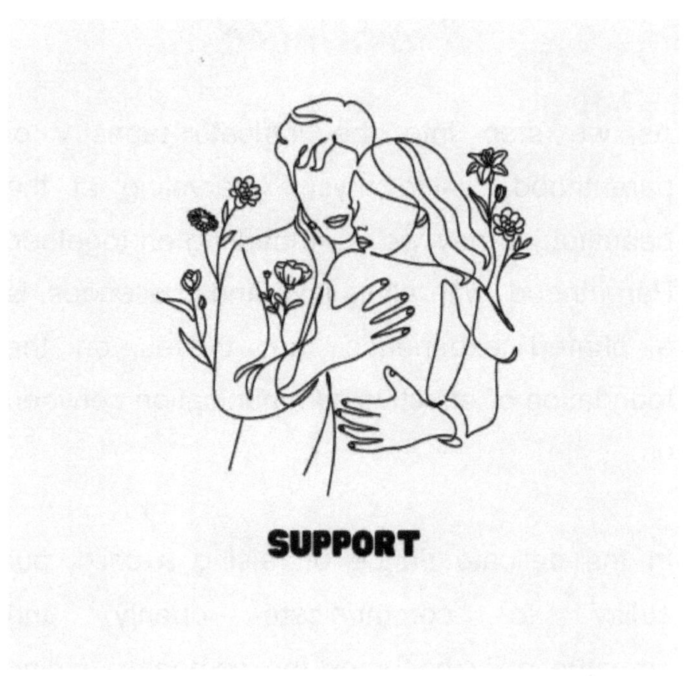

i . Communication in Parenthood

As we step into the intricate tapestry of parenthood, I find myself marveling at the beautiful journey we're embarking on together. Parenthood, with all its joys and challenges, is a shared experience that thrives on the foundation of effective communication between us.

In the delicate dance of raising a child, our ability to communicate openly and empathetically becomes the compass guiding us through the twists and turns of this incredible journey. It's not just about the words we exchange but the understanding, support, and shared decisions that unfold in the dialogue between us.

One of the fundamental aspects of our communication is the distribution of responsibilities. As we navigate the demands of childcare, household tasks, and the intricacies of our individual work commitments, an open conversation about how we can share these responsibilities ensures that neither of us feels overwhelmed. Let's continuously revisit and revise these roles, ensuring that they align with ur strengths and preferences. Parenthood brings with it a spectrum of emotions and challenges. Regular check-ins about how we're feeling, both individually and as a team, become touchstones that ground us in the present moment. Let's actively listen and empathize with each other's perspectives, creating a space where our thoughts and emotions can be freely expressed and understood.

Decision-making is a collaborative process that shapes our parenting journey. From choosing childcare options to making decisions about our child's education, our ability to communicate and make choices together reinforces a sense of shared responsibility. Let's ensure that decisions are not made unilaterally but are products of our collective insights and values.

Flexibility is the glue that holds our parenthood journey together. Unexpected situations and challenges are inevitable, and our ability to communicate openly about changes in routines or unexpected hurdles allows us to adapt gracefully. Let's be each other's pillars of support as we navigate the twists and turns of parenting life.

Expressing our needs and expectations is a continuous conversation that evolves with the changing dynamics of parenthood. Whether it's a need for some alone time, assistance with specific tasks, or emotional support, being transparent about our needs fosters an environment of understanding and support. Regular check-ins on each other's needs ensure that our support strategies are always aligned.

As we venture into this journey, let's approach it as a team. Discussing our parenting goals, values, and aspirations creates a united front in raising our child. In moments of challenge, let's be each other's cheerleaders, recognizing and appreciating the unique contributions each of us brings to our shared role as parents.Disagreements are a natural part of any partnership, and establishing healthy communication patterns for resolving conflicts is crucial. Let's focus on finding solutions rather than assigning blame, using "I" statements to express our feelings and needs. In the face of disagreement, let's remember that we are allies, not adversaries.

Quality time together, as partners and not just parents, is a nourishing ingredient in our relationship. Despite the demands of parenthood, let's consciously carve out moments for connection and relaxation. These moments strengthen our emotional connection and remind us of the bond we share beyond the roles of mom and dad.

Celebrating each other's achievements in parenting, whether big or small, is an essential practice. Positive reinforcement not only acknowledges our efforts but strengthens the bond between us. Let's express gratitude for the energy, time, and love each of us invests in parenting and maintaining our family.

If ever the need arises, let's be open to seeking professional support. Whether it's couples counseling or parenting classes, these resources can enhance our communication skills, offering tools and insights that strengthen our partnership.

As we embark on this extraordinary journey of parenthood, I'm grateful for the partnership we share. Our ability to communicate openly, support each other, and face the challenges

with a united front is the bedrock upon which
our family's story unfolds.

ii. Sharing Responsibilities

Sharing responsibilities in a partnership, particularly in the context of parenthood, is not just about dividing tasks but is deeply intertwined with supporting each other. When both partners actively contribute and collaborate in various aspects of family life, it fosters a sense of shared commitment, strengthens the bond between them, and creates a supportive environment. Here's how sharing responsibilities relates to supporting each other:

1. Equitable Workload:

   - Sharing responsibilities ensures that the workload is distributed fairly. This helps prevent one partner from feeling overwhelmed or burdened by the demands of parenthood and household duties.

   - A balanced workload contributes to a more harmonious partnership, allowing both individuals to maintain their well-being and energy levels.

2. Mutual Understanding:

- Actively participating in shared responsibilities promotes a deeper understanding of each other's daily challenges, commitments, and priorities.

- Understanding the intricacies of your partner's responsibilities fosters empathy, as both individuals recognize and appreciate the efforts invested in different aspects of family life.

3. Team Approach:

- A shared responsibility mindset transforms parenting into a team effort. This collaborative approach strengthens the sense of unity and partnership.

- Working together as a team creates a supportive environment where challenges are faced collectively, and victories are celebrated together.

4. Emotional Support:

- Actively sharing responsibilities is an expression of emotional support. It communicates a commitment to navigating the ups and downs of parenthood together.

- The emotional support derived from sharing responsibilities reinforces the idea that both partners are in this journey together, providing a sense of security and connection.

5. Flexibility and Adaptability:

- Shared responsibilities allow for flexibility and adaptability in addressing the evolving needs of family life. When both partners are actively involved, it becomes easier to adapt to unexpected situations or changes in routines.

- Flexibility is a key component of support, as partners can navigate challenges more smoothly when they collaborate and adjust together.

6. Strengthening the Partnership:

- Sharing responsibilities nurtures a sense of interdependence, where both partners contribute to the overall well-being of the family.

- This interdependence strengthens the partnership, creating a foundation of trust, reliance, and mutual respect.

7. Time for Connection:

- When responsibilities are shared, it frees up time for both partners to connect on a personal level. Quality time together becomes more achievable, enhancing emotional intimacy.

- This connection is vital for maintaining a strong emotional bond, which in turn contributes to a supportive and fulfilling partnership.

8. Encouraging Individual Growth:

- Shared responsibilities allow each partner to contribute their unique strengths and skills. This encourages individual growth and a sense of fulfillment.

- Supporting each other's personal and professional development becomes more feasible when responsibilities are shared, as both partners have the opportunity to pursue their interests and goals.

In essence, sharing responsibilities is not only a pragmatic approach to managing the demands of family life but also a profound expression of mutual support. It reinforces the idea that both partners are active participants in shaping the family's journey, and it lays the groundwork for a resilient and supportive partnership.

iii. Emotional Support

Supporting yourselves emotionally as expectant parents is crucial during this transformative period. The emotional well-being of both partners contributes to a positive and connected pregnancy experience. Here are some ways to foster emotional support:

1. Open Communication:

- Foster open and honest communication about your feelings, expectations, and concerns. Create a safe space for both partners to express themselves without judgment.

2. Attend Prenatal Classes Together:

- Participate in prenatal classes to gain insights into childbirth, baby care, and postpartum adjustments. This shared knowledge can strengthen your bond and ease anxieties.

3. Seek Guidance and Information:

 - Educate yourselves about pregnancy and parenting. Understanding the changes happening during pregnancy can alleviate uncertainties and empower both partners.

4. Share Responsibilities:

 - Collaboratively share responsibilities related to pregnancy preparations, such as attending doctor's appointments, setting up the nursery, and researching baby care essentials.

5. Connect with a Supportive Community:

 - Join prenatal groups, either in-person or online, to connect with other expectant parents. A spirit of support and camaraderie can be fostered by exchanging experiences and guidance.

6. Prioritize Self-Care:

- Both partners should prioritize self-care. Whether it's taking time for hobbies, relaxation, or self-reflection, maintaining individual well-being contributes to a healthier emotional state.

7. Express Feelings About Parenthood:

- Share your thoughts and emotions about impending parenthood. Acknowledge any fears, excitement, or uncertainties and discuss how you can support each other through these emotions.

8. Create Rituals and Bonding Moments:

- Establish rituals or bonding moments that are meaningful to both of you. This could be taking evening walks, reading to the baby, or attending prenatal yoga classes together.

9. Plan for Quality Time:

- Be intentional about spending quality time together. As the due date approaches, prioritize moments that nurture your connection and allow for relaxation and enjoyment.

10. Be Flexible and Manage Expectations:

- Recognize that each pregnancy is unique, and emotional experiences can vary. Be flexible in adapting to changes and manage expectations by embracing the unpredictability of this transformative journey.

11. Seek Professional Support if Needed:

- If emotional challenges become overwhelming, consider seeking professional support. A therapist or counselor specializing in prenatal and postpartum mental health can provide guidance.

12. Practice Mindfulness and Relaxation Techniques:

- Explore mindfulness practices or relaxation techniques, such as meditation or deep breathing exercises. These can help manage stress and promote emotional well-being.

13. Encourage Emotional Expression:
- Create an environment where both partners feel comfortable expressing their emotions. Whether through talking, writing, or other forms of expression, encourage the sharing of feelings.

14. Establish a Support System:
- Be in the company of a network of friends and family who are there to support you. Having individuals who understand and respect your emotional needs can be invaluable.

Remember, supporting yourselves emotionally is an ongoing process. By fostering open communication, seeking knowledge, and prioritizing self-care, expectant parents can navigate the emotional landscape of pregnancy together, creating a foundation for a healthy and connected family.

PART 2

Labor and Delivery

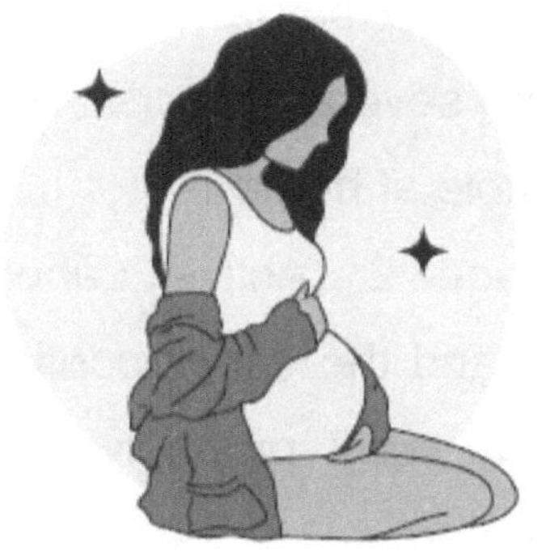

i. Understanding the Process

Understanding the labor and delivery process is essential for expectant parents as it helps alleviate anxieties and allows for better preparation. Here are key aspects to consider:

1. Stages of Labor:

-Stage 1 (Early Labor): Contractions begin, and the cervix starts to dilate. This stage can last for several hours and is typically manageable at home.

-Stage 2 (Active Labor): Contractions intensify, and the cervix continues to dilate. At this point, you'll probably visit a hospital or birthing centre.

- Stage 3 (Delivery of the Baby): The baby is born during this stage.

-Stage 4 (Delivery of the Placenta):The placenta is delivered after the baby.

2. Signs of Labor:

   - Recognize signs of labor, including regular and increasingly intense contractions, the release of the mucus plug, and the rupture of the amniotic sac (water breaking).

3. Labor Positions:

   - Understand different labor positions, as movement and changing positions can help ease pain and facilitate the birthing process. Positions like squatting, kneeling, or standing may be explored.

4. Pain Management Options:

   - Familiarize yourself with pain management options, ranging from natural methods (breathing techniques, movement) to medical interventions (epidural, analgesics). Talk to your healthcare practitioner about your preferences.

5. Role of the Birth Partner:

- Discuss and establish the role of the birth partner during labor. Whether it's providing emotional support, assisting with comfort measures, or advocating for your preferences, their involvement is crucial.

6. Birth Plan:

- Develop a birth plan outlining your preferences for labor and delivery. Share this plan with your healthcare team but remain flexible as circumstances may require adjustments.

7. Monitoring and Interventions:

- Understand common monitoring procedures during labor, such as electronic fetal monitoring. Be aware of potential interventions like induction or assisted delivery methods (forceps, vacuum extraction).

8. Breathing Techniques:

- Practice breathing techniques for labor. Techniques like slow, deep breaths during contractions can help manage pain and promote relaxation.

9. Cervical Dilation and Effacement:

- Learn about cervical dilation (opening of the cervix) and effacement (thinning of the cervix), as these are key indicators of labor progress.

10. Movement and Massage:

- Explore movement and massage techniques to alleviate discomfort. Walking, swaying, or receiving massages from your birth partner can provide relief during labor.

11. Perineal Massage:

- Consider perineal massage techniques to reduce the risk of tearing during delivery. Discuss this with your healthcare provider and seek guidance on proper methods.

12. Episiotomy:

- Understand the concept of episiotomy (a surgical cut to widen the vaginal opening) and discuss its necessity and alternatives with your healthcare provider.

13. Skin-to-Skin Contact:

- Familiarize yourself with the benefits of immediate skin-to-skin contact with your baby after delivery. Discuss this preference with your healthcare team.

14. Postpartum Care:

- Learn about postpartum care, including what to expect immediately after delivery and in the days following. Understand the importance of rest and self-care during the postpartum period.

15. Unexpected Situations:

- Be aware that labor and delivery may not always go as planned. Familiarize yourself with potential complications and trust your healthcare team to guide you through unexpected situations.

16. Hospital Policies:

- Understand the policies of the hospital or birthing center where you plan to deliver. This includes visitor policies, COVID-19 protocols, and any specific guidelines they may have.

17. Postpartum Mental Health:

- Recognize the importance of postpartum mental health. Understand common postpartum emotions and seek support if needed. Communicate your feelings with your partner.

18. Childbirth Education Classes:

- Consider taking childbirth education classes, either in person or online, to gain comprehensive knowledge and practical tips for labor and delivery.

Remember, every labor and delivery experience is unique. Stay informed, communicate openly with your healthcare team, and be flexible in your approach. Trust in your ability to adapt and navigate this transformative process with the support of your partner and healthcare professionals.

ii. Creating Birth plan

As you embark on the incredible journey of preparing for labor and delivery, crafting a birth plan can be a valuable tool to articulate your preferences and create a roadmap for the birthing experience. A birth plan is a reflection of your hopes, desires, and expectations during this transformative process. Let's delve into the considerations and elements to encompass as you create a comprehensive birth plan.

Begin by fostering open communication with your healthcare provider. Initiate a dialogue about your birth plan early in your pregnancy, ensuring that both you and your provider are on the same page regarding your preferences and the options available to you. This collaborative approach establishes a foundation of trust and shared decision-making.

Consider the environment in which you envision bringing your baby into the world. Whether you prefer a calm and dimly lit room, the presence of specific individuals, or your favorite music playing softly, communicate these preferences. Detail the ambiance that will make you feel most comfortable during labor and delivery.

Outline your preferences for pain management, recognizing that your choices may evolve during labor. Whether you opt for natural pain management techniques, epidural anesthesia, or a combination of both, ensure your healthcare team is aware of your preferences and the circumstances under which you would consider alternative options.

Discuss and decide on the birthing positions you find most comfortable. Whether it's standing, squatting, or utilizing a birthing stool, expressing your preferences empowers you to actively participate in the birthing process. Be open to the possibility of movement and changes in positions to navigate the intensity of contractions.

Address the use of medical interventions, such as continuous fetal monitoring, episiotomy, or assisted delivery methods. Clearly communicate your stance on these interventions, and discuss under what circumstances you would be comfortable considering them. Being informed about the potential benefits and risks allows you to make decisions aligned with your preferences.

Consider your wishes for the immediate postpartum period. If you desire immediate skin-to-skin contact with your baby, delayed cord clamping, or specific newborn procedures, express these preferences. Discuss the feasibility of these requests with your healthcare team and explore how they can be accommodated.

Incorporate your choices for the delivery of the placenta, whether you prefer a natural process or the use of interventions. Discuss your preferences for the administration of Pitocin to reduce bleeding and the potential need for manual extraction.

Outline your preferences for postpartum care, including your desire for rooming-in with your baby, breastfeeding support, and any specific cultural or spiritual practices you wish to incorporate into the immediate postpartum period.

While crafting your birth plan, remain flexible. Recognize that unforeseen circumstances may arise, requiring adjustments to your original preferences. Trust in the expertise of your healthcare team and foster open communication to make informed decisions as the situation unfolds.

Lastly, share your birth plan with your healthcare provider and the members of your birthing team well in advance of your due date. Discuss the plan during prenatal visits to ensure clarity and alignment with the practices of the birthing facility.

In creating your birth plan, remember that it is a dynamic document, subject to adjustments based on the progress of labor and individual circumstances. Your birth plan serves as a guide, a shared vision of the birthing experience that can enhance communication and contribute to a positive and empowered journey into parenthood.

Wishing you a safe and fulfilling birthing experience.

iii. partners role in Labour

As we stand on the threshold of one of the most significant moments in our lives, partners presence during the upcoming labor and delivery must be deeply felt. In this journey, your role is not just supportive; it's fundamental to the very essence of this transformative experience.

Emotional support is a beacon of strength during labour. In the midst of labor, your calming presence, reassuring words, and comforting touch create an environment of security and encouragement. Your positivity has the power to shape the atmosphere of the birthing room, making it a sanctuary of love and support.

You play a vital role as an advocate for our shared desires and birth plan. Understanding our preferences for pain management, birthing positions, and postpartum practices, you are to become the voice that communicates our wishes to the healthcare team. Your role as an advocate ensures that our choices are considered and respected throughout the process.

In the realm of physical comfort, your touch becomes is a source of solace during contractions. Whether it's a gentle massage, helping change positions, or providing counterpressure, your physical support becomes an anchor during the intensity of labor.

As a communication liaison between your partner and the healthcare team, you hold a crucial position. Your role is to facilitate clear communication, ask questions on our behalf, and keep us well-informed about the progression of labor and any potential interventions. Your active involvement in this dialogue ensures that we make decisions collaboratively.

Familiarizing yourself with birthing positions, you guide through different postures that feel comfortable, providing encouragement during these changes. Your involvement in exploring these positions becomes an integral part of the birthing process.

Staying informed about the stages of labor, potential interventions, and the birthing environment, you become a steady and knowledgeable presence. Your calm demeanor and collected approach in understanding the unfolding events contribute to a sense of assurance during the intensity of labor.

Your role extends into the postpartum period. Beyond the birthing experience, your support with tasks, assistance with immediate postpartum care, and attentiveness to both my needs and those of our newborn create a seamless transition into the next phase of our journey.

In moments where appropriate, your capturing of photographs or videos becomes a beautiful way to document the essence of this monumental experience. These captured moments will be cherished for a lifetime, telling the story of our journey into parenthood.

navigating through this unpredictable and miraculous process, your flexibility and adaptability become guiding principles. Your ability to go with the flow, adjust to changing circumstances, and maintain a positive attitude contributes immensely to the overall experience.

As the arrival of the little one approaches, Your role is not just witnessed in actions but felt in the depth of shared emotions. Together, you will navigate labor and delivery as a united team, welcoming little ones into the world.

PART 3

Bringing Baby Home

i. Postpartum Adjustments

As you embark on the postpartum journey, it's important to recognize that this period brings about a series of adjustments as you settle into your new roles and responsibilities. Here are some aspects to consider and navigate during this transformative time:

1. Physical Recovery:

   - Allow yourself time for physical recovery after childbirth. Your body has undergone significant changes, and it's crucial to prioritize rest, proper nutrition, and gentle exercise as recommended by your healthcare provider.

2. Emotional Well-Being:

   - Be attuned to your emotional well-being. Hormonal changes, sleep deprivation, and the demands of caring for a newborn can contribute to a range of emotions. Seek support from your partner, friends, and family, and don't hesitate to communicate openly about your feelings.

3. Sleep Deprivation:

- Understand that sleep patterns will be disrupted with a newborn. Create a flexible sleep routine that allows both parents to share responsibilities, and take naps whenever possible to manage fatigue.

4. Establishing Routines:

- Gradually establish routines for feeding, diapering, and sleep. Predictability can provide a sense of stability for both you and your baby.

5. Partner Support:

- Lean on your partner for support. Share responsibilities, communicate openly about your needs, and work together to navigate the challenges of parenting.

6. Seeking Help:- Ask for help from friends, family, or professionals when needed. Accepting assistance can alleviate the workload and provide you with moments of respite.

7. Changes in Relationship Dynamics:

   - Recognize that your relationship with your partner may undergo adjustments. Communication is key. Discuss the changes you're experiencing, express your needs, and find moments to connect amidst the demands of parenthood.

8. Emotional Rollercoaster:

   - Understand that postpartum emotions can be a rollercoaster. It's normal to experience moments of joy, frustration, and even moments of doubt. Seek emotional support and communicate openly with your partner.

9. Postpartum Body Image:

- Embrace the changes in your body. It took time to grow and nurture your baby, and it will take time for your body to readjust. Be patient with yourself and focus on self-care.

10. Postpartum Check-ups:

- Attend your postpartum check-ups with your healthcare provider. Discuss any concerns or questions you may have about your physical or emotional well-being.

11. Bonding with Baby:

- Nurture your bond with your baby through skin-to-skin contact, talking, and spending quality time together. Building a strong connection is an ongoing process.

12. Time for Yourself:

- Carve out moments for self-care. Whether it's a brief walk, a quiet moment with a book, or a warm bath, prioritize time for activities that bring you comfort and relaxation.

13. Patience with Adjustments:

- Understand that adjustments take time. The postpartum period is a phase of learning and adapting. Be patient with yourself and your partner as you navigate this new chapter in your lives.

Remember, there's no one-size-fits-all approach to postpartum adjustments. Each family's journey is unique. Be open to adapting strategies that work best for you, and surround yourself with a supportive network to navigate the joys and challenges of this transformative time.

ii. Newborn Care Basics

Congratulations on the arrival of your precious little one! As you embark on this incredible journey of parenthood, here are some newborn care basics to help you navigate the initial weeks and create a nurturing environment for your baby:

1. Feeding:

   - If you're breastfeeding, ensure a comfortable latch and feed on demand. If formula feeding, follow guidelines for preparing and feeding formula. Aim for frequent feeds, especially in the first weeks.

2. Diapering:

   - Change diapers regularly, about every 2-3 hours or as needed. To avoid diaper rash, keep the diaper region dry and clean. Use a gentle diaper cream if necessary.

3. Bathing:

- Sponge bathe your newborn until the umbilical cord stump falls off. Use mild baby soap and shampoo, and be gentle when handling your baby. After the stump falls off, transition to gentle tub baths.

4. Sleep:

Generally sleeping 16–17 hours a day, newborns sleep for long periods of time. Create a safe and comfortable sleep environment, placing your baby on their back to sleep. Follow the ABCs of safe sleep: Alone, on their Back, in a Crib.

5. Swaddling:

- Swaddling can provide comfort and promote sleep. Use a light, breathable blanket to swaddle your baby snugly, ensuring their hips can move freely.

6. Clothing:

- Dress your baby in soft, comfortable clothing. Make sure the temperature is just right for them. A good rule of thumb is to add one extra layer to what you're wearing.

7. Bonding:

- Spend quality time bonding with your baby through skin-to-skin contact, talking, and making eye contact. Respond promptly to your baby's cues, and enjoy these precious moments of connection.

8. Tummy Time:

- Start tummy time from day one to help strengthen your baby's neck and upper body muscles. Begin with short sessions and gradually increase as your baby becomes more comfortable.

9. Pacifiers:

- Pacifiers can offer comfort to a fussy baby and may reduce the risk of Sudden Infant Death Syndrome (SIDS) when used during naps and bedtime.

10. Baby Gear Safety:

- Always follow safety guidelines for baby gear, such as car seats, strollers, and cribs. Ensure that your baby's sleep space is free from loose bedding, toys, and other potential hazards.

11. Regular Check-ups:

- Make an appointment for routine check-ups with your paediatrician to track your child's development and growth. Keep track of vaccinations and discuss any concerns you may have.

12. Crying:

- Babies cry as a way of communicating. Attend to your baby's needs by checking for hunger, diaper changes, tiredness, or discomfort. If your baby continues to cry, seek comfort measures and consult your pediatrician if needed.

13. Parental Self-Care:

- Make self-care a priority for both you and your relationship. Adequate rest, proper nutrition, and emotional support are essential for both parents during this adjustment period.

Remember, every baby is unique, and there is no one-size-fits-all approach to newborn care. Trust your instincts, seek guidance when needed, and savor the special moments with your new boundle of joy.

iii. Sleep and Self-Care Tips

Congratulations on navigating the whirlwind of parenthood! As you embark on this rewarding journey, it's crucial to prioritize your well-being, especially when it comes to sleep and self-care.

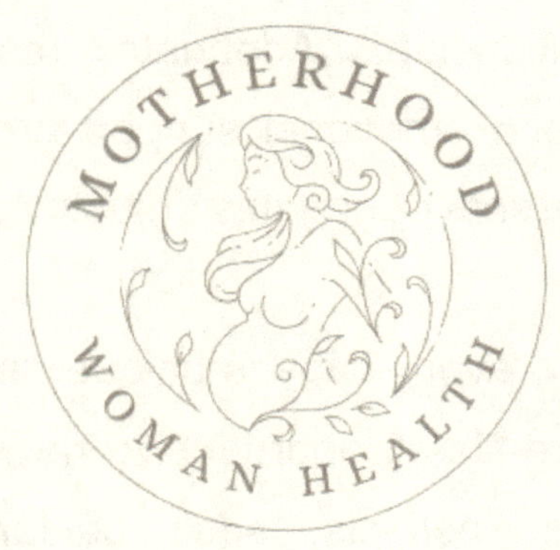

Here are some tips to help you catch those much-needed and carve out moments for yourself amidst the joys and demands of parenting:

1. Embrace the Power of Naps:

   - When your baby naps, consider taking a nap yourself. Even short power naps can make a significant difference in restoring your energy levels.

2. Create a Consistent Sleep Environment:

   - Create a relaxing nighttime ritual to let your body know when it's time to relax. Dim the lights, engage in relaxing activities, and create a comfortable sleep environment.

3. Sleep When Your Baby Sleeps:

   - It's a classic piece of advice for a reason. Take advantage of your baby's nap times to grab some extra sleep for yourself. The laundry or dishes can wait – your well-being is a priority.

4. Accept Help:

- Accept assistance from friends and relatives without hesitation. Whether it's someone watching the baby while you nap or taking care of household tasks, accepting support can alleviate the load.

5. Prioritize Self-Care Rituals:

- Identify self-care activities that bring you joy and relaxation. Whether it's a warm bath, reading a book, or enjoying a cup of tea, schedule regular moments for self-care.

6. Set Realistic Expectations:

- Understand that your sleep patterns may be disrupted during the early months of parenthood. Set realistic expectations and be patient with yourself as you adapt to the new normal.

7. Share Responsibilities:

- Collaborate with your partner to share responsibilities, especially during nighttime awakenings. Consider taking turns soothing the baby or handling night feedings to ensure both parents get adequate rest.

8. Limit Screen Time Before Bed:

- Reduce exposure to screens before bedtime. Electronic device blue light can disrupt the production of melatonin, making it more difficult to fall asleep.

9. Stay Hydrated and Nourished:

- Maintain a healthy diet and stay hydrated. Proper nutrition contributes to overall well-being and can impact your energy levels.

10. Establish a Relaxing Bedtime Routine:

- Develop a bedtime routine for yourself. Engage in activities that promote relaxation, such as gentle stretching, reading, or practicing mindfulness.

11. Communicate Your Needs:

   - Communicate openly with your partner and loved ones about your sleep and self-care needs. Establish a support system that understands the importance of your well-being.

12. Delegate and Let Go:

   - Delegate tasks and be willing to let go of perfection. Your well-being is more important than having a spotless home. Prioritize what truly matters.

13. Consider Professional Support:

   - If sleep deprivation becomes overwhelming, consider seeking professional support. A sleep consultant or therapist specializing in postpartum issues can provide guidance and strategies.

Recall that caring for oneself is a need, not an extravagance. By prioritizing sleep and incorporating self-care into your routine.

Wishing you resilience, joy, and moments of profound connection in your postpartum journey.

Conclusion

it's essential to recognize that the path ahead is both joyous and demanding. Through the sleepless nights and tender moments, remember that taking care of yourself is not only a gift to you but also to your little one.

In the whirlwind of diaper changes, lullabies, and the sweet scent of baby lotion, don't forget to prioritize your well-being. Sleep, that elusive treasure, may come in fragments, but each moment of rest is a step towards rejuvenation. Embrace the beauty of naps, create a soothing sleep environment, and, most importantly, be kind to yourself as you navigate the unpredictable terrain of parenthood.

Self-care isn't a luxury; it's a vital component of being the best parent you can be. Whether it's stealing a quiet moment for a cup of tea, indulging in a favorite book, or simply breathing in the stillness, these small acts of self-nurturing have the power to replenish your spirit.

As the days unfold, communicate openly with your partner, seek support when needed, and accept the helping hands extended by friends and family. Remember that parenthood is a shared journey, and through collaboration and understanding, you'll weather the challenges and relish the triumphs together.

In conclusion, embrace the messy, beautiful chaos of parenthood with an open heart. Cherish the sleepless nights, revel in the tiny victories, and allow self-care to be a constant companion on this transformative adventure. May each day bring you closer to the profound joy that comes with watching your little one grow and thrive.

Wishing you boundless love, enduring patience, and moments of pure bliss as you navigate this extraordinary chapter in your life.